ALL YOU WANTED TO KNOW ABOUT
HIV and AIDS

Edited by
Dr Savitri Ramaiah

New Dawn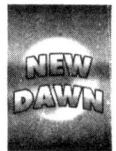

NEW DAWN
An imprint of Sterling Publishers (P) Ltd.
A-59 Okhla Industrial Area, Phase-II, New Delhi-110020.
Tel: 6387070, 6386209   Fax: 91-11-6383788
E-mail: ghai@nde.vsnl.net.in
www.sterlingpublishers.com

All You Wanted to Know About - HIV and AIDS
© 2000, Sterling Publishers Private Limited
ISBN 81 207 2304 x
Reprint 2002

All rights are reserved. No part of this publication may be reproduced, stored in a retrieval system or transmitted, in any form or by any means, mechanical, photocopying, recording or otherwise, without prior written permission of the publisher.

Published by Sterling Publishers Pvt. Ltd., New Delhi-110016
Lasertypeset by Vikas Compographics, New Delhi-110029.
Printed at VMR, New Delhi.

Information for this series, has been provided by *Health Update*, a monthly bulletin of the Society for Health Education and Learning Packages. The Update is intended to provide you with knowledge to adopt preventive measures and cooperate with the doctor during illness for better outcome of treatment.

Contributor

ALLOPATHY
Dr Vijaya Srinivasan
(Director, Gandhigram Institute of Rural Health and Family Welfare Trust, Gandhigram, Dist. Dindigul, Tamil Nadu)

Preface

All You Wanted to Know About is an easy-to-read reference series put together by *Health Update* and assisted by a team of medical experts who offer the latest perspectives on body health.

Each book in the series enhances your knowledge on a particular health issue. It makes you an active participant by giving multiple perspectives to choose from — allopathy, acupuncture, ayurveda, homoeopathy, nature cure and unani.

This book is intended as a home adviser but does not substitute a doctor.

The opinions are those of the contributors, and the publisher holds no responsibility.

Contents

Preface   4
Introduction   9
What is HIV/AIDS?   13
What is the history of HIV/AIDS?   15
What is the structure of HIV?   19
How does HIV affect the body?   23
How does HIV spread in the body?   25
How common is HIV/AIDS?   31
How does HIV/AIDS spread?   36
What are the symptoms of HIV/AIDS?   67
What are the opportunistic infections in AIDS?   78
How is HIV diagnosed?   84
When is a blood test for HIV recommended?   91

When should treatment for HIV infection be started?	94
What is the treatment for HIV infection?	99
How is the benefit of the treatment assessed?	112
What is the role of other systems of medicine management of HIV infection?	114
What are the dietary recommendations for HIV infection?	121
What is the risk of occupational exposure to HIV?	125
What is the treatment for occupational exposure to HIV?	128
How can HIV/AIDS be prevented?	133
What are the benefits of using condoms?	135

What are the different types of condoms?	139
How can diseases be prevented in people with HIV infection?	141
How can mother-to-child transmission of HIV infection be prevented?	162
How is HIV infection in children diagnosed?	167
What are the symptoms of children with HIV infection?	169
What is the progress of HIV infection in children?	171
Is there a vaccine to prevent HIV infection?	173
What are the ethical issues related to HIV infection?	174

Introduction

Few diseases have been feared as much as HIV/AIDS has been ever since human beings began efforts to prevent and control major diseases. History is witness to several successful attempts of mankind in eradicating, controlling or preventing major causes of death or disability. Eradication of smallpox and control of diseases such as polio, measles, tetanus, etc., through vaccines, etc. are examples of human being's triumph over several killer diseases. Although a large number of health problems continue to defy human efforts to control them, none of them presents a challenge greater than the prevention and control of HIV/AIDS. This is mainly because at the moment there is neither a scientifically proven cure for HIV/AIDS nor a vaccine to prevent it.

Several misconceptions about the causes and mode of transmission of HIV/AIDS exist in India. These misconceptions and the social stigma associated with AIDS have been major barriers to prevent and control the disease. They have also been major hurdles in providing the desirable social and medical support to people with HIV infection.

All predictions related to the spread of HIV infection in India portray a very grave situation unless active measures are taken to prevent and control the infection. In response to this grave threat, several donor agencies such as World Health Organisation, World Bank, United Nations agencies, etc., have provided funds to the Government of India's National AIDS

Control Programme. Several non-governmental and other agencies have been supplementing the government's efforts to control HIV/AIDS in India. Although these efforts have been substantial, much more needs to be done to prevent and control the disease. This book focuses on the history of HIV/AIDS, its mode of transmission, symptoms laboratory investigations, its prevention treatment of HIV infection, opportunistic infections and their prevention. It also describes the current understanding of reducing the risk of mother to child transmission of HIV infection. The main purpose of discusing HIV/AIDS in detail is to help you understand the disease process better, and with the hope that you will use this understanding to educate people about its preventive measures and provide support to those who are living with HIV infection. Every individual effort can go a long way in preventing the rapid spread of HIV/AIDS in India and helping those living with HIV lead a life with dignity.

What is HIV/AIDS?

HIV is the abbreviated form of Human Immuno-deficiency Virus. This virus causes Acquired Immuno Deficiency Syndrome or AIDS. Thus, HIV is the name of the virus and AIDS is the name of the disease. As the name AIDS implies, it is a condition where there is deficiency in the body's natural defence mechanism or the immune system. It is "acquired" because it is not a *hereditary* condition or due to long-term use of some medicines, such as those for treatment of cancer. Hereditary means conditions that are passed on from one generation to another. This means that AIDS is acquired because of certain behavioural patterns. *Syndrome* means a group of symptoms. When one gets AIDS, there can be a wide range of symptoms, all of which are due to the body's diminished ability to fight diseases.

It is important to remember that everyone who has HIV infection will develop AIDS over a period of time depending upon their general health and natural defence mechanism of the body.

What is the history of HIV/AIDS?

As mentioned earlier, HIV/AIDS is a relatively new health problem. In 1981, several medical practitioners in USA were puzzled because a large number of young men were developing *pneumonia* due to a new type of bacteria or a rare type of skin cancer called *Kaposi's sarcoma*. Both these diseases were earlier observed only in people with damaged natural defence mechanism (immune system) of the body. In addition, these patients had several other infections also. Pneumonia is the term used for inflammation of the lungs due to any disease-causing agent. The most common cause of pneumonia is the bacteria called *pneumococcus*.

Initially, symptoms of pneumonia and kaposi's sarcoma were observed only in homosexual men, but soon they were found in other sections of the society such as those with *haemophilia* or those who were *intravenous* drug users. Haemophilia is a hereditary disease where the blood lacks some essential components necessary for clotting of blood and healing of wounds. Intravenous means injecting a substance into the veins. Thus, the medical practitioners concluded that the disease spread through sexual route among the homosexuals and blood route among the intravenous drug abusers or those requiring regular transfusion of blood or blood products.

By 1982, it was evident that a new disease had emerged. During this time, doctors in Africa also came across people with unusual symptoms. It soon became evident that the new disease in the USA and Africa were one and the same. The virus that caused the disease was first identified and isolated independently in 1984 by scientists in France and the US. This new virus was called HIV in 1986. Subsequently, one more virus was identified which was also capable of producing signs and symptoms of AIDS. The virus, first isolated was called HIV-1 and the virus identified later was called HIV-2.

The origin of HIV viruses and AIDS is still a mystery. There have been three main theories about its origin but none of them have been proven so far. In fact all of them have limitations. The first theory is that the HIV existed in a small isolated community and was somehow transmitted to the outside world. The second theory is that it may have been transmitted from an animal, such as monkey. The third theory is that some existing viruses may have changed their genetic structure and therefore developed a new variety of the virus. It is important to remember that all the three theories have several deficiencies and therefore the origin of HIV remains unknown. Also, understanding the origin of the virus may not contribute significantly in developing strategies to prevent and control HIV infection.

What is the structure of HIV?

Just as all viruses, the HIV is also a very small infectious particle that can be seen only through an electron microscope. The virus is so small that when about ten thousand viruses are put together in a circle, they will have a diameter of about one millimetre!!!! Figure 1 illustrates the structure of HIV virus.

It consists of an outer coating of fat. This fat layer has two types of special particles — GP-120 and GP-41. GP is the short form for *glyco-protein*, which means a sugar containing protein. GP-120 helps the virus to first attach itself to the cells and then attack them. GP-41 also plays a role when the virus is ready to attack the cells. Below the fat layer containing glyco-proteins are

Figure 1. Structure of Human Immuno-deficiency Virus

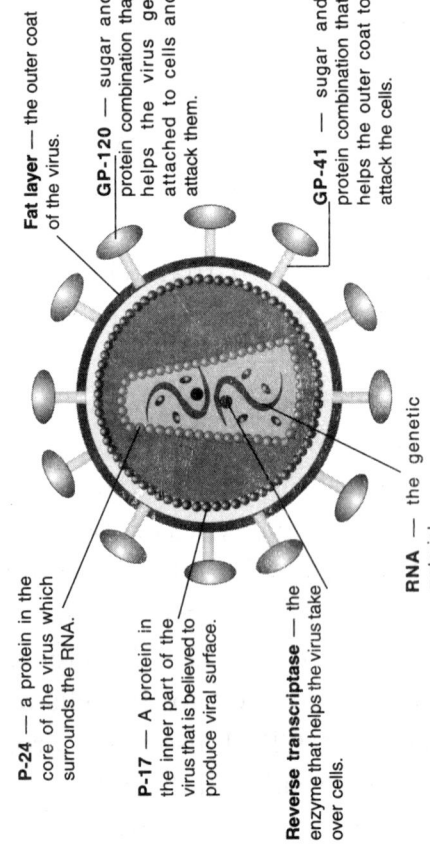

Fat layer — the outer coat of the virus.

GP-120 — sugar and protein combination that helps the virus get attached to cells and attack them.

GP-41 — sugar and protein combination that helps the outer coat to attack the cells.

P-24 — a protein in the core of the virus which surrounds the RNA.

P-17 — A protein in the inner part of the virus that is believed to produce viral surface.

Reverse transcriptase — the enzyme that helps the virus take over cells.

RNA — the genetic material

two protein layers called P-24 and P-17. P-17 is the protein in the inner shell and is suspected to produce the surface of the HIV. P-24 is the core protein and it surrounds two strands of RNA, which is the short form for *ribonucleic acid*. The RNA is normally present in the central part of the cell called "nucleus" and its surrounding part called the "cytoplasm". It transmits the instructions from the nucleus to the cytoplasm. In the cytoplasm, the RNA mainly assembles proteins.

Each strand of RNA in the HIV contains a copy of nine *genes*, which are the biological units of genetic material and inheritance. Three of these nine genes contain information necessary to make proteins for new viruses. The other genes contain information necessary for the production of proteins that are important for their ability to infect a cell, produce new copies or cause disease. At the end of each strand of RNA is an enzyme called *"reverse transcriptase"*. This enzyme helps the HIV to take over the human cells.

How does HIV affect the body?

HIV destroys a particular variety of white blood cells that are essential for destroying disease-causing germs. There are several varieties of white blood cells in the body. Of these, *lymphocytes* form about twenty-five per cent of the total white blood cell count. They normally increase in number in response to any infection. There are two types of lymphocytes: (a) B cells and (b) T cells. When the B cells come in contact with a disease-causing agent such as bacteria or virus, they secrete large volumes of *antibodies* — chemical substances that can destroy the disease-causing germs. The main functions of B cells are to search, identify and then bind with the disease-causing germs.

The T cells are lymphocytes that have travelled through a small gland called the *thymus gland*, which is situated in the middle and upper part of the bony cage of the chest. When a disease-causing germ enters the body, the T cells produce several new copies of itself. Each T cell contains chemical substances that can destroy the specific disease- causing germs. T cells are also called "killer cells" because of their two main actions, which are (a) they secrete chemical substances necessary for destroying the disease-causing germs and (b) they help the B cells in destroying the agents.

How does HIV spread in the body?

There are six steps through which the HIV multiplies and affects the cells. These are illustrated in Figure 2 and described in detail below.

1. *Entry of HIV into cells:* Some cells of the immune system contain a molecule called CD4 on their surface. CD4 molecules are also found on the T cells. When the HIV virus enters the body, it first identifies cells with CD4 and attaches itself to them. Once the HIV binds with the CD4, the membranes of the virus and the T cell fuse. As a result of this fusion, the virus's RNA, proteins and enzymes enter the T cell. It is

Figure 2. Process of infection of a human cell by HIV

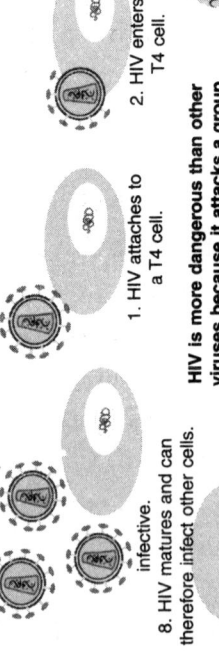

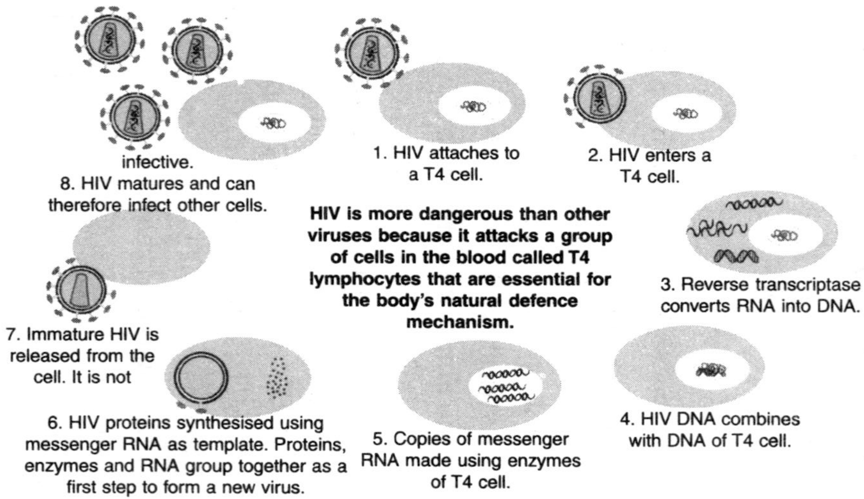

1. HIV attaches to a T4 cell.

2. HIV enters a T4 cell.

3. Reverse transcriptase converts RNA into DNA.

4. HIV DNA combines with DNA of T4 cell.

5. Copies of messenger RNA made using enzymes of T4 cell.

6. HIV proteins synthesised using messenger RNA as template. Proteins, enzymes and RNA group together as a first step to form a new virus.

7. Immature HIV is released from the cell. It is not infective.

8. HIV matures and can therefore infect other cells.

HIV is more dangerous than other viruses because it attacks a group of cells in the blood called T4 lymphocytes that are essential for the body's natural defence mechanism.

important to remember that although the main target for HIV is the T cells, it also attaches itself to other types of white blood cells containing CD4 but does not destroy them. These cells can act as reservoirs of HIV if the natural defence mechanism of the body tries to destroy the HIV.

2. *Reverse transcriptase:* Once the RNA, proteins and enzymes of the HIV enter the cytoplasm of the T cell, an enzyme called, *"reverse transcriptase"* present in HIV converts RNA into DNA, which is an abbreviated form of deoxyribonucleic acid. DNA is a form of nucleic acid that carries genes, the basic unit of genetic inheritance.

3. *Integration:* In this stage, the newly-formed DNA of the HIV enters the T cell's nucleus and is incorporated into

its genes. Thus, when the T cell multiplies, the virus DNA is also copied. A person infected with HIV may contain billions of cells containing the HIV DNA.

4. *Transcription:* The T cell that contains HIV/DNA cannot produce new viruses unless the RNA is able to make its own copies. It is important that these RNA are "read" by the protein- making mechanism of the infected T cell. To enable production of RNA copies and therefore to allow multiplication of new viruses, a special type of RNA called *"messenger RNA"* is produced. The process of production of messenger RNA is called transcription. This process involves the enzymes of the infected T-cell. The genes of HIV and the protein-making mechanism of the

T cells together control the process of transcription.

5. *Translation:* After the messenger RNA of the HIV is processed by the nucleus of the infected cell, it is sent in to the cytoplasm. In the cytoplasm, the virus collaborates with the T cell's protein-making mechanism to make long chains of proteins and enzymes of HIV. The messenger RNA acts as a template or guide for production of HIV proteins and enzymes. The process of making long chains of viral proteins and enzymes is called translation.

6. *Assembly and budding:* In this stage, the newly made HIV proteins, enzymes and RNA collect *just inside* the wall of the infected T cell. At the same time, the proteins that form the covering of the virus collect *within the wall* of the infected T cell. Next, an immature

particle of the virus is formed and it separates from the infected T cell. This new viral particle has an envelope that includes proteins from the walls of both, the HIV and the infected T cell. It is important to remember that the immature virus cannot spread the infection to other people.

The long chains of proteins and enzymes formed inside the infected cell are cut into smaller pieces by a specific enzyme of the virus called *protease*. This step results in formation of viral particles that can spread infection to other T cells.

How common is HIV/AIDS?

Since 1981, when the first case of AIDS was reported in the United States, AIDS has spread all over the world and has become a major public health problem in several countries. An estimated 23 million people worldwide are reported to be living with the HIV infection. All of them will develop AIDS within the next ten years. About eighty thousand people worldwide are estimated to be infected with the HIV infection per day.

Ninety per cent of people with HIV infections are in the developing world, and of these the majority are in Sub-Saharan Africa. As per the estimates of the World Health Organisation, about thirty to forty million people all over the world will be infected by HIV by the next year and of these eight to ten million people will develop AIDS.

The first AIDS case in India was reported in 1986 from Chennai. Since then there has been a rapid spread of HIV infection all over the country. By March 1998, the National AIDS Control Organisation had reported that a total of seventy-one thousand four hundred people were having HIV infection from among 3.2 million people who were tested for it. During the same period, a total of five thousand one hundred forty-five people had been reported to have had developed AIDS. Of these, about eighty per cent were males and twenty per cent females. Almost eighty-nine per cent people with AIDS were in the age group of fifteen to forty-four years, which are the most economically productive years for any individual.

Maharashtra has reported the maximum number of HIV infections followed by Tamil Nadu and Manipur. *Sentinel Surveillance* reports from various parts of the country have shown varied rates of HIV infection. Sentinel surveillance involves (a) choosing a limited number of population groups and sites where these groups can be accessed and (b) testing a sample of individuals in these sites on a systematic basis, such as once in a year. Normally, sentinel groups are those where blood samples are routinely collected for some specific blood tests. During the period when the surveillance is planned, HIV testing is done for the sentinel groups in addition to the blood tests routinely done for them. This type of surveillance ensures that the blood tests can be done conveniently and anonymously. Thus, the names of the people who were tested for HIV infection are not recorded.

In India, the sentinel groups are (a) people attending special clinics for sexually transmitted diseases, (b) intravenous drug users and (c) pregnant women consulting with a doctor for routine check-up. The first two groups are high-risk groups for HIV and therefore give an early warning to an approaching *epidemic*. Epidemic is the term used for a condition where a significantly large number of people are affected with the same health problem at the same time. The pregnant women represent a general population, which is typically at lower risk, and indicates how much the epidemic has spread beyond the high-risk groups. Sentinel surveillance has indicated that 4.6 per cent to 36 per cent people attending sexually transmitted diseases' clinics, 32 per cent to 85.6 per cent people using intravenous drugs and 0.5 per cent to 4.25 per cent pregnant women have HIV infection.

How does HIV/AIDS spread?

HIV infection spreads through four main routes: (a) sexual transmission, (b) blood transfusion, (c) injections, especially intravenous drug injections and (d) mother-to-child transmission during pregnancy or delivery. Figure 3 shows the probable source of HIV infections and AIDS in India. More than seventy-four per cent people are estimated to have got the infection through sexual transmission.

The effectiveness of transmission of the virus by various routes is not the same. Effectiveness of transmission means the chance or probability of getting the infection with one encounter with the virus through that route. The effectiveness is often expressed as percentage. This means

Figure 3. Probable sources of infection in AIDS in India

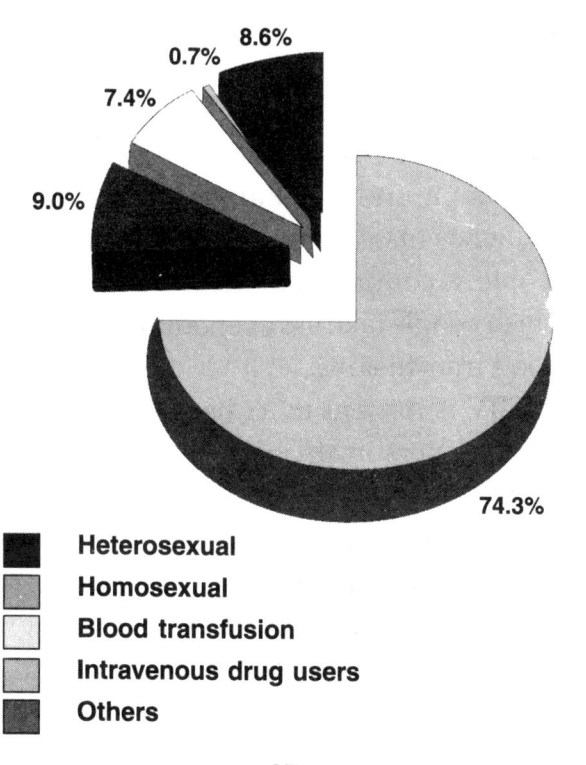

- Heterosexual — 74.3%
- Homosexual — 9.0%
- Blood transfusion — 7.4%
- Intravenous drug users — 0.7%
- Others — 8.6%

the number of times a person can get HIV infection through exposures to the route of transmission. Box 1 shows the effectiveness of transmission by various routes. It is important to remember that although sexual route has a very low effectiveness of transmission, it accounts for more than seventy-four per cent infections in India. This is mainly because of the high frequency of occurrence of sex acts among people as compared to the frequency with which people take intravenous drugs or get blood transfusions.

HIV is present in all body fluids of an infected person. It is, however more in number in blood, *semen* and *vaginal fluids*. Semen is the thick whitish secretion of the male reproductive organs that is discharged from the same opening through which the urine comes out. Vaginal fluids are the secretions from the *vagina*, which is a like a canal in the female reproductive system. It starts at the opening of the womb or uterus, and opens out of the body just behind the opening for urine and in front of the opening for stool. HIV virus can be easily killed by heat and by drying. Four main conditions must be fulfilled if HIV is to be transmitted through any one of the four routes mentioned above. These include:

1. HIV must be present in the body fluids, especially the semen, vaginal fluids, blood.
2. HIV must live during the period it is out of the body. It can live for a long time in blood stored at cold temperatures for transfusion but lives for a very short time in all other situations as the body fluids dry easily. HIV cannot survive in dried body fluids.

Box 1. Effectiveness of transmission of HIV infection by various routes

- Needles and syringes — 70%
- Blood transfusion — 90-95%
- Sexual route — Less than 1%
- Mother to baby — 40%

3. There must be a convenient place for the virus to enter the body. The normal skin forms a very effective barrier against HIV and will find it difficult to enter the body through intact skin. The virus can easily enter the body from where there is either damage to the skin or the skin is more delicate (such as in vagina or the *anus*). Anus is the opening of the digestive tract through which stool is passed out of the body.
4. The number of viruses in the body fluids must be adequate to infect others after it is transferred on contact with body fluids. If the number of viruses that enter another person is less, the infection may not occur.

Detailed below are the critical issues related to each of the four above modes of transmission of HIV.

Sexual transmission: The most common route of spread of HIV infection is through unprotected sex between two people, one of who has HIV infection. Unprotected sex means having sex without a condom. Unprotected vaginal sex, where the *penis* is inserted into the vagina is more common source of infection in India as compared to unprotected anal sex where the penis is inserted into the anus. Penis is the external reproductive organ of a man. HIV is present in the *sperms* as well as the *seminal fluids*. Sperms are the mature male "seeds" or the germ cells. When a sperm "unites" with the female egg (ovum), fertilisation occurs. Seminal fluid is thick, whitish secretions of the male reproductive organs that is discharged from the body during ejaculation.

Even one episode of unprotected sex with an infected partner can transmit HIV.

The risk of HIV being transmitted from an individual sexual act depends upon several factors. Increased number of unprotected sex with an infected partner increases the risk of infection.

Women are at a greater risk of developing HIV infection through unprotected sex. This means that the risk of transmission of HIV from man to woman is higher than that from woman to man. There are several reasons why women are at greater risk.

1. The semen from the infected male sexual partner remains in the woman's vagina for a longer time. Longer contact between infected semen and the delicate outer wall of the vagina increases the risk of HIV infection.

2. The surface area of the vagina is very large compared to the urethra in men, the opening through which semen and

urine is passed out of the body. Larger surface area provides greater opportunity for the virus to enter the body.

3. A large number of women who have infections of their reproductive tract may not have any symptoms at all. In the absence of any symptoms, women will not know they have the infections and will therefore not take appropriate treatment. These infections allow greater opportunity for the HIV to enter the body and cause infection.

Some important factors that help transmission of HIV infection are detailed below and summarised in Box 2.

Sexually transmitted diseases: Any ulcer, injury or damage to the outer wall of the penis or vagina can increase the risk of getting HIV infection. Several sexually transmitted diseases cause ulcers or sores

Box 2. Factors that help transmission of HIV infection

- **Sexually transmitted diseases** increase the risk of HIV infection because they allow easy entry for the HIV in the body.
- **Anal sex**, irrespective of whether it is between a man and a man or a man and a woman increases the risk of HIV. This is because the delicate skin inside the anus gets damaged more easily during the sexual act.
- **Sex during menstruation** with a woman having HIV infection increases the risk of transmitting HIV to the male partner.
- **Oral sex** has low risk of transmission of HIV. The risk is higher in case there are wounds, cuts or injuries in the mouth.
- **Blood transfusion** has a small risk of transmitting HIV. Although the government has made testing the blood for HIV before

transfusion compulsory, the test may be negative up to 3-6 months after getting the infection.

- **Intravenous drug injections** have a very high risk of transmission of HIV especially among drug abusers who share needles to inject addictive drugs. Intravenous injection with sterilised needles and syringes have no risk of transmitting HIV.
- **Pricking the skin** for tattooing, piercing ears, nose, etc., have low risk of transmitting HIV infection if sterilised needles are used.
- **Pregnant women** can transmit the HIV infection to their unborn child either during pregnancy or during childbirth.
- **Breast-feeding** has low risk of transmitting HIV infection to the baby. The risks of bottle-feeding are higher than the risks of HIV infection due to breast-feeding. This is why it is recommended that women with HIV infection continue to breast feed their baby.

on the penis or walls of the vagina. The HIV can therefore easily enter the body through the damage to the genital skin caused by these ulcers and sores. Also, the whitish secretions due to sexually transmitted diseases contain large number of white blood cells. Large number of white blood cells mean large number of the virus in this pus. Since increased number of viruses in the body fluids increases the risk of transmitting HIV infection, a person with sexually transmitted diseases has a higher risk of transmitting HIV infection to the sexual partner.

Anal sex: This is the term used when the penis is inserted into the anus of the sexual partner. Although anal sex is more common among homosexuals, a large number of heterosexual partners also practice it. Anal sex has a higher risk of transmitting HIV infection as compared to vaginal sex. This is mainly because the inner lining of the anus is delicate and therefore gets damaged very easily during anal sex. This damage helps the HIV to enter the body and cause infection.

Homosexual sex: This is the term used when people prefer to have sex with partners of their own sex. Until recently, cultural taboos had prevented people from talking about homosexuality openly. Increased awareness about HIV/AIDS has resulted in more and more people willing to talk about homosexuality. Several studies have indicated that the number of homosexual males is higher in India that what was thought to be until a few years ago. A large number of homosexual males in India are married and have children. They therefore consider themselves as heterosexual people who have occasional sex with male partners. Majority of the sexual partners of eunuchs (*hijras*) are men. Although there are several people who are homosexual in India, HIV infection has not been widely reported among them. The main route of transmission of HIV continues to be heterosexual sex. This does not mean that there is low risk of getting HIV infection through homosexual sex in India. It means that at present there is higher risk in heterosexual sex mainly because people practising heterosexual sex is far more than those practicing homosexual sex.

Female homosexual sex (called lesbianism) is considered to have a very low risk of spreading the HIV infection. This is mainly because homosexual sex among women is non-penetrative.

Menstruation: The menstrual blood of a woman with HIV infection will contain the virus. Thus, sexual intercourse during menstruation with an infected woman increases the risk of the male partner getting HIV infection.

Blood transfusions: You are at no risk of getting HIV infection when you donate blood. This is because the needle and other equipment used for collecting your blood is normally disposable and therefore safe. However, people who get blood transfusion that is infected with HIV have a very high risk of getting HIV infection. The risk of getting HIV infection due to blood transfusion is almost nil in the developed countries such as the US and Europe. This is mainly because of compulsory blood testing for HIV infection before it is transmitted.

Although the National AIDS Control Organisation in India has made testing of blood for HIV before transmission mandatory, some medical experts believe that there is a small risk of transmitting HIV infection through blood transfusion. This is mainly because the blood tests normally done to detect HIV infection in India can identify only the *antibodies* against HIV. Since the body requires about three to six months to produce antibodies, the HIV test is likely to be negative up to three to six months after getting the infection. Since a person can transmit HIV even before the blood tests indicate the presence of antibodies, there is a low risk of transmitting HIV infection through blood transfusion in India. This risk can increase if there is high level of HIV infection in the general population. Given the several risks involved with blood transfusion (HIV is just one of them), most medical practitioners prefer to give blood transfusion only if there is an emergency and it is essential to preserve life.

In India, blood transfusion is normally given after surgery or accidents when there is excessive loss of blood and severe anaemia due to a wide range of causes. *Thalassaemia* is one of the important causes of anaemia in India. In this condition, regular blood transfusions are essential for survival. Thalassaemia is a hereditary condition where there is a deficiency in the synthesis of haemoglobin. Since haemoglobin carries oxygen to different parts of the body, defective production of haemoglobin will lead to reduced oxygen carrying capacity of the blood.

Haemophilia is another hereditary disease in which the blood does not clot in case of any injury. Thus, there is risk of excessive bleeding even after minor injuries. People with haemophilia regularly require a substance called *Factor VIII*, which is prepared from the blood. When the HIV infection was first detected, many people got infected worldwide because of the virus present in Factor VIII. In recent years, the blood used to prepare Factor VIII is given heat treatment so that the HIV gets killed. Factor VIII is therefore not a potential source of HIV infection anymore.

Intravenous injections: When people inject drugs intravenously, they may draw small amount of blood into the needle. If another person uses this needle immediately, the blood containing HIV will be injected into the second person. Thus, he/she can also be infected with HIV. Normally, people who are addicted to intravenous drugs form a group and share needles with each other. Thus, the infection can spread very rapidly from one to another in the same group. In India, intravenous drug abuse is the most important cause of HIV infection in Manipur.

Intravenous injections are sometimes necessary for management of several health problems. In case the health care provider has not sterilised the needles properly, and it had been used for a person who had HIV infection, there is a risk of spreading HIV infection to others. It is, however, important to remember that despite several reports about poor quality of health care delivery services in India, HIV infection through injections given at a health centre is not a common mode of transmission. This is mainly because HIV is destroyed by heat and drying. A large number of health professionals prefer to use disposable needles and syringes, thereby avoiding the risk of transmitting HIV. Some medical practitioners, especially those in rural areas who have not been trained in medical schools are reported to be practising poor sterilisation of needles and syringes. They however, boil them for a short time, which is adequate to kill HIV. Shorter boiling time for sterilising needles may not destroy other disease causing germs such as Hepatitis B virus. It is also important to remember that injections that are given in the muscles, under the skin or in the skin layers carry little risk of transmitting the HIV. They however can carry higher risk of transmitting infections such as Hepatitis B.

In recent times, there have been rumours that a some people who have HIV infection intentionally prick other people with infected needles in public places such as movie theatres, markets, bus-stops, etc., and therefore transmit the infection to them. These rumours are baseless. There are several reasons why the infection is not likely to be transmitted in this way. One, there should be adequate amount of blood containing the virus on the needle before it can cause infection. A needle that has been merely pricked in the body of a person with HIV is not likely to have the number of HIV necessary to cause infection. Two, even if the infected person were to use needle that has been used intravenously, the virus may not be alive if the blood on the needle has dried up. Three, when an infected needle is pricked into the muscles, the risk of transmitting the infection is very low.

Mother-to-child transmission: HIV can cross the *placenta* from the mother to the infants before birth. Placenta is a flat cake-like organ that has a large number of blood vessels. The unborn baby in the mother's womb receives oxygen and other nutrients through the placenta and excretes carbon dioxide and other wastes through the placenta.

HIV infection can also be transmitted to the baby during delivery. About thirty to thirty-five per cent babies born to women who have HIV Infection are likely to be infected also. A child born to a mother who has AIDS is more likely to get HIV infection.

Some studies have indicated that HIV is present in the breast milk. This is why some medical practitioners recommend that women with HIV infection avoid breast-feeding the newborn baby. However, this recommendation is not universally acceptable. Although HIV is present in the breast milk, it does not mean that the baby will always be infected with it. Also, in a country such as India, the alternative to breast-feeding is bottle-feeding. This is not only expensive but also carries a higher risk of diarrhoea, poor nutrition and as a result death. Since the benefits of breast-feeding are much more than the risk of getting HIV infection, medical practitioners in India strongly recommend that all women with HIV infection should breast-feed their babies.

Skin piercing: There are several cultural practices in India that involve skin piercing. These include piercing ears or nose for ornamental reasons, tattooing, circumcision, etc. At the moment, skin piercing is not one of the major routes of transmission of HIV infection in India. However, if the number of people with the infection were to increase in the general population, the risk is likely to be higher. This is why it is important to ensure that the equipment used for skin piercing is sterilised well. A large number of people prefer to get ears and nose pierced by traditional goldsmiths than medical professionals. Irrespective of the current level of risk, it is important to ensure that the instruments used by them are sterilised as per the recommended guidelines.

Oral route: Some studies have persuasively indicated that HIV is present in the saliva and other body fluids. This is why many people believe that kissing, sharing utensils, etc., with people who have HIV can transmit the infection. This is not necessarily true. The concentration of HIV in the saliva is very low and it therefore carries a very low risk of transmitting the infection. Also, it is believed that the chemical substances in the saliva can destroy the HIV. If the virus is ingested in the stomach, the acids in it are likely to inactivate or destroy the virus. The risk through oral route is therefore very low. It can be higher if there are cuts or wounds in the mouth or bleeding gums. This is because the blood that oozes out of the mouth will have HIV.

There are several misconceptions about the spread of HIV infection through oral sex. Some studies have indicated that oral sex has a higher risk of transmitting HIV infection as compared to kissing. This is because oral sex allows vaginal secretions and/or semen to enter the mouth. In case there are wounds or injuries in the mouth, the virus present in vaginal secretions or semen can easily enter the body. Although the risk of getting HIV infection is lower with oral sex if there are no wounds in the mouth, it is not recommended as an alternative to safer sex, i.e., sex using a condom.

Box 3 lists the routes through which HIV infection cannot be transmitted.

Mosquito bites: Many people believe that since mosquito bites transfer blood from one person to the another, it can also spread HIV infection from an infected person to others. This is however not true. The amount of blood that a mosquito sucks while biting a person is very small. Thus, even if the virus were to enter the mosquito's body, the number of viruses will be too less to cause infection in others. Also, the HIV virus does not live outside human fluids. Mosquitoes can spread diseases such as malaria because the malarial parasite multiplies in the body of the mosquito and increases the number of parasites that can infect other people. HIV does not multiply outside the human body and therefore cannot increase in number in the mosquito's body.

Box 3. Ways in which HIV does not transmit

- Hugging
- Kissing
- Shaking Hands
- Kissing on the cheeks, hands, etc.
- Coughing or sneezing
- Insect bites
- Sharing clothes
- Sharing towels
- Using the same equipment such as telephone
- Eating from the same utensils
- Swimming pools
- Sharing the same toilets
- Being with infected people in a crowd or public places
- Mosquito bites
- Nursing people with HIV infection
- Washing clothes, bed spreads, etc., used by people with HIV infection

Medical and paramedical professionals: People in medical and paramedical professions often come in contact with body fluids of infected people. This is why some people believe that those in these professions are at a higher risk of getting HIV infection. If the recommended precautions are taken, such as using double gloves, avoid performing surgeries — both minor and major — when they have cuts or injuries in their hands or any other body part that is likely to come in contact with the patient, medical and paramedical professionals can prevent the transmission of infection. The World Health Organisation has recommended a set of precautions for medical and paramedical professionals for prevention of HIV infection. These precautions are called Universal Precautions against HIV infection transmission. Regular practice of these precautions can protect these professionals.

Guidelines for universal precautions are listed in Box 4.

Box 4. Guidelines for universal precautions

- Universal precautions need to be practised at all times, as it is difficult to say who has HIV infection just by looking at them.

- Wear gloves if there is a risk of contact with blood and body fluids either while examining a person or doing any other procedure.

- Wear eyeglasses or goggles, mask and gown if there is risk of the body fluids or blood splashing on you.

- Always wash hands before and after physical contact with a patient.

- Always wash hands after removing the gloves.

- For washing hands, use running water for at least half a minute.
- Liquid soap is preferable to solid soap for washing hands.
- Use 0.5-1 per cent sodium hypochlorite solution to disinfect surface that have come in contact with body fluids or blood.
- Use waterproof dressings to cover cuts or abrasions during physical contact with the patient.
- Do not pass sharp instruments hand-to-hand. Place them in a flat surface so that the other person can pick it up.
- Do not use hand needles.
- Do not guide needle into the body of the patient with the fingers.
- Do not reheat the needles.

What are the symptoms of HIV/AIDS?

A person infected with HIV is not likely to have any symptoms for about three to ten years. This period may be longer if the natural defence mechanism of the body is good. As mentioned earlier, although a person infected with HIV does not have any symptoms, he/she can spread the infection to others. This is why it is recommended that anyone who has sex with a partner who is not in mutually faithful relationship should practice safe sex. This means using a condom correctly for every sexual act.

In order to understand why HIV infection does not cause symptoms for a long time, it is important to understand the events that take place in the body soon after

HIV enters it. As mentioned earlier, HIV infects a large number of CD4 cells soon after it enters the body. It multiplies rapidly in the T4 cells that contain CD4 particles. During the early or acute stage of the infection, the blood will contain a large number of viral particles. These particles rapidly spread through various organs and infect several organs of the body. They particularly infect the organs of the *lymphatic system.*

Lymphatic system is a vast, complex network of capillaries, thin vessels, ducts, valves and organs. This entire network helps to protect and maintain the internal fluids of the body. They do this by producing, filtering and transporting *lymph* to various parts of the body. Lymph is a thin clear fluid that is produced by various organs of the body and is circulated in the lymphatic network. It enters the bloodstream in the large veins of the neck.

There are small nodes called lymph nodes in the lymphatic system. They filter the lymph and fight infection. Various types of blood cells essential for fighting infection are formed in the lymph nodes.

The effect of HIV infection on the lymphatic system results in decrease in the total number of CD4 and T cells in the bloodstream by twenty to forty per cent. Two to four weeks after the first entry of the virus in the body, up to seventy per cent people suffer flu-like symptoms related to acute infection. The symptoms may be fever, headache, enlarged lymph nodes and a general feeling of being unwell. All these symptoms are often mild and not very specific. This is why it is difficult to differentiate symptoms due to HIV infection from those of other viral infections. By the time the flu-like symptoms appear, the normal defence mechanism of the body fights back with the killer T cells and the antibodies produced by B cells. As a result, the HIV levels in the body reduce dramatically and the total number of CD4 and T cells may go back to eighty to ninety per cent of the original levels.

After the active stage of multiplication and the body's response to the virus, a person infected with HIV will not have any symptoms for several years. During this time, the HIV continues to multiply in the organs of the lymphatic system. Most scientists believe that this is because after the initial activity of the T cells where they kill the HIV, they seem to exhaust themselves and disappear. In the absence of the killer cells, HIV continues to multiply. Also, the killer T cells tend to accumulate in the blood whereas the HIV is largely located in the lymphatic system.

As mentioned earlier, people with HIV infection do not develop persistent severe symptoms for up to ten years after the virus first enters the body. Children born with HIV infection may however develop the symptoms within two years. The symptoms appear because of the gradually diminishing defence mechanism of the body. This is the stage when AIDS develops. Most symptoms of AIDS are due to opportunistic infections that take advantage of the body's poor defence mechanism. Opportunistic infections are those infections that may not cause disease in a person with normal defence mechanism.

The symptoms of AIDS are divided into major and minor symptoms. As per the definition of AIDS given by the World Health Organisation, a person is said to have AIDS if he/she has at least two major signs and at least one minor sign and there is no other cause of poor immune mechanism. The term *"AIDS related illness"* is used when a person has some of the signs and symptoms, has antibodies to HIV in the blood but does not have two major and one minor sign.

Detailed below are the major and minor signs and symptoms that are listed in Box 5.

Major signs: Diarrhoea is very common in people with AIDS. It is normally clear and watery and may be associated with cramp-like pain in the abdomen and vomiting. Chronic diarrhoea with excessive loss of weight is one of the important features of AIDS. There may also be

Box 5. Signs and symptoms of AIDS

Minor signs:
- Persistent cough for more than one month.
- Enlargement of the lymph nodes in various parts of the body.
- Fungal infection of the mouth or throat called oral candidiasis or thrush.
- Dermatitis: Itchy skin lesions all over the body
- Recurrent infections of herpes zoster, a viral infection that results in painful and small eruptions on the skin along a nerve affected by the virus.
- Chronic herpes simplex, another viral infection that affects the skin and the nervous system. It results in small, transient, irritating and sometime painful fluid filled blisters on the skin and mucous membrane — thin sheet of tissue that lines the cavities and canals of the body that open outside, such as mouth, respiratory tract, urinary, etc.

Major signs:
- Unexplained loss of weight, greater than ten per cent of the total body weight during one month.
- Chronic fever that lasts for more than one month.
- Chronic diarrhoea that lasts for more than one month.

continuous fever and increased sweating at nights.

Minor signs include chronic cough that does not respond to routine treatment, enlargement of the lymph nodes, fungal infection of the mouth called candidiasis, recurrent infections of herpes group of viruses.

- *Enlarged lymph nodes:* As mentioned earlier, the lymph nodes are essential for maintaining the body's normal defence mechanism. They are located in groups in various parts of the body such as armpits, neck and groin. Enlarged and painless lymph nodes in various parts of the body is one of the early signs of AIDS. It is important to remember that any infection can cause enlarged lymph nodes. Normally, only those lymph nodes located near the affected part of the body are enlarged. In case of an infection that affects the entire body, lymph nodes all over the body get enlarged.

- *Fungal infection of the mouth:* One of the common symptoms of AIDS is an infection in the mouth called candidiasis. This is due to a yeast called candida. Candidiasis results in a thick, white and fur-like coating on the tongue and roof of the mouth. It can also cause dry mouth, difficulty in swallowing, and an altered sense of taste. This infection is not common among people with normal defence mechanism because their body is able to fight the infection successfully.

Candidiasis may also be present in old people with poor defence mechanism, sick children and babies who are fed by bottles. It can also affect the vagina in women. Candidiasis in people with AIDS can also spread to the lungs and the digestive tract.

- *Fungal infection of the lungs:* Pneumocytis carnii pneumonia is a fungal infection of the lungs that results in symptoms similar to the pneumonia due to bacterial infection. It results in persistent dry cough and death can occur when it spreads to other parts of the body.
- *Infection due to herpes viruses:* Herpes simplex and herpes zoster are two common viral infections in people with AIDS. Herpes simplex can affect anyone, but it is more severe in people with AIDS. It produces small blisters filled with fluids that may be painful. These sores occur more often inside and

around the mouth, genital area or the area around the anus. The sores of herpes simplex in people with normal defence mechanism lasts for about two to three days and are few in number. They last longer and are more in number in people with AIDS.

Herpes zoster is also a viral infection that starts as a painful rash with blisters. These rashes are more common on the face, trunk and limbs. If they affect the eyes, pain and blurring of vision may occur. Herpes zoster is normally seen in old people who have poor defence mechanism. In recent years, it has become more common in young people with AIDS.

What are the opportunistic infections in AIDS?

Poor defence mechanism of the body allows several disease-causing germs to infect people with AIDS. Detailed below are some of the common opportunistic infections seen in people with AIDS.

Tuberculosis: This is a bacterial infection and is normally transmitted when a person with active tuberculosis coughs or sneezes. During the act of coughing or sneezing, germ particles of tuberculosis called *droplet nuclei* are released in the air. These droplet nuclei contain the bacteria that cause tuberculosis. When a healthy person inhales the droplet nuclei, he/she can get infected with tuberculosis. Many people in India who are infected with tuberculosis develop *latent infection* only. Latent infection means the infected person will neither have any signs or symptoms nor will be able to spread the infection to others. They can however, become sick and get infected with active tuberculosis at a later stage.

Tuberculosis often occurs in the early stages of HIV infection. Since tuberculosis is already one of the major health problems in India, people with HIV infection are at a higher risk of getting it. Very often, tuberculosis is the first indication that a person has HIV infection. Although tuberculosis largely affects the lungs, it can affect other organs of the body also. People with AIDS are more likely to get infection in other organs of the body.

One of the major concerns related to tuberculosis and AIDS is resistance of the tuberculosis bacteria to several medicines that were earlier effective for its treatment. Resistance of medicines normally occurs when people fail to complete a course of treatment. Since treatment for tuberculosis takes several months, there is a very high rate of drop-outs. People who fail to complete the full course of treatment can become resistant to medicines and spread the resistant bacteria to others also. Resistant tuberculosis is one of the important causes of early death in people with HIV infection.

Tuberculosis is more common in people with HIV infection who have less than two hundred CD4+ count.

Common symptoms of tuberculosis include cough, fever, increased sweating at nights, loss of weight and excessive fatigue.

AIDS dementia complex: This is not a true opportunistic infection. It is one of the few conditions caused directly by the HIV virus. HIV can cross the blood barrier present all around the brain. It can damage not only the brain but also the spinal cord — the main nerve that emerges from the base of the neck and passes through the backbone — and the nerves.

Common symptoms of AIDS dementia complex include confusion, depression and a strange unusual behaviour. There may be general loss of interest in the surroundings, indifference, etc. In later stages, it causes loss of memory, uncoordinated movements, or paralysis.

Diagnostic diseases: Kaposis's sarcoma and cryptococcal meningitis are the two diseases that are a definite indication of AIDS.

- *Kaposis's sarcoma:* This is the most common cancer seen in people with AIDS. Some studies have indicated that this cancer is due to infection by one of the herpes groups of viruses. Some other studies have indicated that it is due to an abnormality of the production of blood cells. Although more studies are necessary to identify the cause of kaposis's sarcoma, its presence is a definite indication of AIDS.

Common symptoms of kaposis's sarcoma include red or purple raised areas on the skin. They may also be present in internal organs of the body such as mouth, lymph nodes, digestive tract and lungs. Recent advances in management of kaposis's sarcoma have increased the chances of complete recovery.

- *Cryptococcal meningitis:* This infection is caused by a yeast-like fungus called *cryptocossus neoformans*. It is found in soil in most parts of the world, especially the soil that is contaminated with bird droppings. In the early stages of the infection, the fungus affects the brain and the lungs. In later stages, it can affect any other part of the body. Cryptococcal meningitis is more common among people with CD4 count less than fifty.

Common symptoms of cryptococcal meningitis include fever, mild headache followed by nausea, vomiting, severe headache and blurring of vision.

How is HIV diagnosed?

There are three main types of tests for testing the blood for HIV infection. These include tests to (a) detect antibodies; (b) identify HIV itself and estimate the number of HIV virus in the body; and (c) provide an estimate of the number of T cells in the blood. Of these three types, the most common are the tests to detect antibodies. Detailed below are the tests in each of these categories:

- ***Tests to detect antibodies:*** The most common test to detect HIV antibodies is the *ELISA test*, which is a short form for Enzyme Linked Immune Assay. ELISA test is preferred as an initial test for HIV testing mainly because it is simple and sensitive. It is therefore suitable for testing large number of blood samples. It is important to remember that there are several ELISA kits available commercially but not all of them have been manufactured using recommended guidelines. It is therefore desirable that the ELISA test be performed in laboratories approved or supported by the National AIDS Control Organisation. These centres use only standard kits.

The Government of India has recommended that a person should be suspected to have HIV infection only if two consecutive and separate ELISA tests have indicated the presence of antibodies. In case the ELISA test indicates presence of antibodies, further tests to confirm HIV infection are recommended. These tests are expensive and therefore many medical practitioners recommend three consecutive

Box 6. What do the HIV test results mean?

Negative test result:
- The person tested does not have HIV infection, or
- The person tested has HIV infection but has not yet made the antibodies against the virus.

Positive test result in a person above 15 months of age:
- The person tested has antibodies against HIV in his/her blood.
- Presence of antibodies indicates that the person has HIV infection. He/She can therefore spread the virus to others.

Positive test result in a person below 15 months of age:
- The child is infected with HIV

    OR

- The child has received antibodies to HIV from his/her mother.
- The HIV antibodies acquired by a child from the mother normally disappear by 15 months.
- HIV test needs to be repeated after the child is 15 months old in order to find out if the child has got the HIV infection or not.

ELISA tests to be done instead of doing a confirmatory test. If each of these tests indicates presence of HIV antibodies, the person is said to have HIV infection.

As mentioned earlier, a person infected with HIV develops antibodies to it only after about three to six weeks. The period between the actual infection and the time when antibodies appear in the blood is called the *window period*. ELISA test will be negative if the blood is tested in the window period.

Other tests to detect antibodies include *rapid tests* such as "dot blot" or "immuno blot", dipsticks, etc., and *simple tests*. These tests are not routinely recommended because of the higher probability of laboratory errors and higher costs as compared to the ELISA tests. Rapid tests give results within fifteen to thirty minutes only. Even if the test result is positive, it is necessary to do ELISA and Western Blot test for confirmation. This is because rapid tests often show false positive results.

Urine and saliva antibody tests have also been developed to detect HIV antibodies in the urine and saliva respectively. Both these tests however do not replace the ELISA test.

The most common test used to confirm HIV infection is the Western Blot test. This test also detects antibodies to HIV. A Western blot test is said to be positive if the test shows reactions to the antigens of at least two of the following components of the virus: P-24, GP-41 and GP-160. A negative test is one which does not indicate antibodies to any of the above components of the virus. In case there is reaction to one or more antigens only, or if there is weak reaction, the test results is said to be doubtful.

It is important to remember that about fifteen per cent people who are not infected with HIV can also have doubtful test result. This is why Western Blot test is recommended only after two consecutive ELISA tests have been positive.

In India, standard ELISA and Western Blot test facilities are available in several major hospitals.

- ***Tests to detect HIV***: The most common test to detect HIV itself is called *polymerase chain reaction or PCR test*. These tests can indicate the presence of the virus in new born babies or adults within a week of their getting HIV infection. The PCR tests can also estimate the number of viruses in the blood and are therefore used to assess the progress of the disease.
- ***Tests to estimate the number of T cells in the blood***: Estimating the number of

T cells in the blood or the total CD4 count in the blood is used for identifying the stage of HIV infection, plan the most suited treatment option and establish the diagnosis of AIDS. It can also be used to decide whether specific preventive measures are desirable for opportunistic infections or not. This is because a decline in CD4 cells indicates increased risk of getting infections.

When is a blood test for HIV recommended?

The HIV test results can have a major impact on the psychological status of the person tested, family, relationship with other members, employment opportunities, etc. This is why HIV testing should not be done without informed consent. This means that the person being tested should understand the consequences of the test results. It is also important to keep the test results confidential. In India, scientifically tested treatment options for people with HIV infection are limited. This is mainly because of the excessive cost. Also, none of the currently available treatment options can cure HIV infection. This is why HIV testing is not routinely recommended even for those who are at a higher risk of getting infected.

HIV testing without consent is done for all blood samples collected for transfusion and during sentinel surveillance. The test results are however confidential and anonymous. Testing the blood for HIV without informed consent is ethically wrong and is strongly discouraged by the Government of India and all agencies involved in prevention and control of HIV/AIDS in India.

It is important to remember that the HIV test does not provide any information to the present state of the person tested. It also does not provide information on the source of infection or whether the infection has been transmitted to others or not.

Since it is not possible to identify people with HIV infection by just looking or interacting with them, and HIV testing is not likely to alter the course of the infection, if any, preventive measures are the only current hope for controlling HIV/AIDS.

When should treatment for HIV infection be started?

The treatment for HIV infection ideally needs to be started as soon as a person gets infected. However, since it is difficult to diagnose HIV infection unless a series of specific blood tests are done, the treatment should start as soon as the infection is detected. People at high risk of getting the infection should be counselled for voluntary testing of blood so that they are able to detect the infection, if any, at the earliest.

The treatment options for HIV infection depend largely on two blood tests:

- *Total number of CD4 or T-cells in the blood:* CD4 or T cells are the cells in the immune system. HIV attacks these cells and destroys them. The normal range for CD4 cells is five hundred to one thousand. Higher the total number of CD4 cells in the blood, better will be the response to treatment for HIV infection.

- *Number of HIV in the body:* There are several tests (such as polymerase chain reaction or PCR) that can estimate the number of HIV in the blood. Lesser the number of the virus in the body better will be its response to the treatment. Estimating the number of HIV in the body not only helps in planning a treatment regime but also helps assess the progress of the treatment. It is important to remember that different methods of estimating the number of virus in the body give different results. This is why only one method of estimating number of virus needs to be used every time the test is repeated. The number of HIV in the body is said to be high if it is more than ten thousand as measured by *DNA test* and more than twenty thousand copies if measured by *PCR assay test*.

Most medical professionals recommend treatment for HIV infection for people in six main categories that are listed in Box 1. There are several other issues related to the decision to start the treatment for HIV infection. These are as described below.

1. The treatment of HIV infection with allopathic medicines proven to be effective is very expensive, often running to more than Rupees two lakhs a year. Few people in India are able to afford these medicines.

2. The treatment is required on long-term basis and it is difficult to ensure

> **Box 7. Criteria for starting treatment for HIV infection**
>
> - Recent HIV infection that has resulted in "flu-like" symptoms.
> - HIV infection of less than six months duration.
> - Presence of opportunistic infections.
> - Less than five hundred CD4 and T cells in the blood or high number of HIV in the blood.
> - The risk of developing AIDS as indicated by the number of HIV in the blood and CD4 cells.
> - Anyone who is willing to accept the treatment regimen and is likely to continue with the treatment schedule.

commitment to follow the treatment schedule strictly for several years.

3. There is a grave risk of severe side-effects of the medicines. Several medicines are contraindicated along with some medicines recommended for other health problems such as

tuberculosis, anxiety, sleep disorders, digestive disorders, etc.
4. The virus can become resistant to one or more medicines, thus making them ineffective.

The above concerns should not prevent a person from seeking treatment if it is accessible and affordable. This is because treatment can prolong life, reduce the rate of progression of the disease and improve the quality of life.

What is the treatment for HIV infection?

Until recently, most medical practitioners recommended only one medicine called *zidovudine* for treatment of HIV infection. However, several studies in recent times have indicated that taking only one medicine increases the risk of the virus developing resistance to it. A combination of two or three medicines is therefore recommended for effective treatment of HIV infection.

Medicines recommended for management of HIV infection can be divided into three groups:
1. Nucleoside Reverse Transcriptase Inhibitors, which are also called NRTIs. These medicines interrupt an early stage

of virus replication. These medicines may slow the spread of HIV in the body and delay the onset of opportunistic infections, however they do not prevent transmission of HIV to other individuals;
2. Non-nucleoside Reverse Transcriptase Inhibitors, which are also called NNRTIs; and
3. Protease Inhibitors, or PIs. These medicines interrupt virus replication at a later stage in its life cycle.

Nucleoside Reverse Transcriptase Inhibitors: There are *five* nucleoside reverse transcriptase inhibitors. Detailed below are their doses and side-effects.

- *Zidovudine (AZT):* This is one of the more commonly used medicines for management of HIV infection. Its recommended dose is two hundred milligrams three times a day or three hundred milligrams twice a day. In recent years, AZT has been recommended in combination with other medicines to control HIV infection.

Common adverse effects include suppression of *bone marrow* (a specialised soft tissue that is present in the bones), anaemia and *neutropenia* (a condition where there is an abnormal reduction in the number of a particular type of white blood cell.) Some people also complain of disturbances in their digestive system, headache, sleeplessness and general weakness.

- *Didanosine:* This medicine is recommended in the dose of two hundred milligrams twice a day for people who weigh more than sixty kilograms and one hundred and twenty-five milligrams twice a day for those who weigh less than sixty kilograms. Common side-effects include nausea, diarrhoea, inflammation of the pancreas and abnormalities in the structure or function of the nerves of the limbs.

- *Zalcitabine:* The recommended dose for this medicine is 0.75 milligrams three times a day. Common side-effects include abnormal structure or function of the nerves of the limbs and swelling of the throat.
- *Stavudine:* Forty milligrams of this medicine is recommended twice a day for people who weigh sixty kilograms or more. For those who weigh less, thirty milligrams is recommended twice a day. Common side-effects include abnormal structure or function of the nerves of the limbs.

- *Lamivudine:* This medicine has the least side-effects and is therefore normally recommended in combination with Zidovudine or AZT. One hundred and fifty milligrams of Lamivudine is recommended for people who weigh more than fifty kilograms. For those who weigh less, the recommended dose is two milligrams per kilogram of body weight.

Abnormal accumulation of *lactic acid* with an abnormal condition of the liver is a rare but potentially life-threatening side effect with the use of all nucleoside reverse transcriptase inhibitors. Lactic acid is a chemical compound that is produced by respiration without oxygen.

Non Nucleoside Reverse Transcriptase Inhibitors: There are *three* main medicines in this group. Detailed below are their recommended doses and their interactions with other medicines.

- *Nevirapine:* Two hundred milligrams of this medicine is recommended four times a day for the first fourteen days followed by the same dose twice a day. Common side-effects include rash, hepatitis and increased levels of an enzyme called *transaminase*.

  Nevirapine interacts with oral contraceptives, some medicines used for treatment of tuberculosis (such as rifampicin), protease inhibitors (recommended for treatment of HIV infection) and triazolam (used for management of sleep disorders including sleeplessness).

- *Delavirdine:* The recommended dose of this medicine is four hundred milligrams three times a day. Common side-effects include rashes and headache. Delavirdine is not recommended with tranquillisers or some medicines used for management of sleep disorders (such as alprazolam, triazolam, midazolam, etc.) medicines used for epilepsy (such as phenytoin, carbamazepine and phenobarbitol), *cisapride* (a medicine used for management of vomiting, increased acids in the stomach) and amphetamines.

Delavirdine increases the level of some medicine such as dapsone (recommended for management of leprosy), clarithromycin (antibiotic), quinidine (used for treatment of malaria) and protease inhibitors such as indinavir and saquinavir (used for management of HIV infection).

Antacids can interact with delavirdine and therefore a gap of about one hour is recommended between taking these two medicines.

- *Efavirenz:* The recommended dose is six hundred milligrams four times a day. Common side-effects include rash, dizziness, sleeplessness, abnormal dreams, confusion, lack of concentration, loss of memory, hallucinations, etc. Efavirenz interacts with medicines such as cisapride, midazolam, triazolam, etc., and is therefore not recommended with them. It also decreases the levels of two protease inhibitors including indinavir and saquinavir and increases the level of two other protease inhibitors including nelfinavir and ritonavir.

Efavirenze can interact with some medicines such as rifampicin, pheynytoin, etc., and is therefore recommended only under direct supervision by a medical practitioner.

Protease inhibitors: There are *four* main types of protease inhibitors. Detailed below are the recommended dosages, interactions with other medicines and the side-effects of protease inhibitors.

- *Indinavir:* Eight hundred milligrams of this medicine is recommended either one hour before meals or two hours after meals. Common side-effects include disturbances of the digestive system. Occasionally some people may have headache, blurred vision, rash, dizziness, metallic taste in the mouth and abnormal bleeding or bruising in the body.

    Indinavir is not recommended with medicines such as rifampicin, cisapride, triazolam and midazolam.

- ***Ritonavir:*** The recommended dose of this medicine is six hundred milligrams twice a day to be taken with meals. This dose is reached by gradually increasing it during fourteen days. The first two days three hundred milligrams of ritonavir is recommended twice day followed by four hundred milligrams twice a day for the next three days. On days six to thirteen, five hundred milligrams is recommended twice a day. Thereafter, six hundred milligrams is recommended twice a day. Ritonavir is often recommended in combination with saquinavir, another protease inhibitor.

Common side-effects include nausea, vomiting, diarrhoea, decreased sensation in the limbs, hepatitis and change in the taste sensation. Ritonavir is not recommended with medicines such as cisapride, tranquillisers, quinidine, etc. It can increase the levels of clarithromycin and decrease the levels of zidovudine.

- *Nelfinavir:* The recommended dose for adults is seven hundred and fifty milligrams three times a day with meals. Common side-effects include diarrhoea, pain in the abdomen, nausea, rashes and increased gas in the bowels. Medicines such as rifampicin, can reduce the levels of nelfinavir. This medicine is not recommended for use along with tranquillisers, cisapride, etc. It increases the levels of other protease inhibitors such as indinavir and saquinavir.

- *Saquinavir:* The recommended dose is six hundred milligrams to be taken three times a day. Some preparations may also be recommended in the dose of twelve hundred milligrams three times a day. Common side-effects include disturbances in the digestive system such as nausea, diarrhoea, pain in the abdomen, headache and indigestion. The levels of saquinavir in the blood are increased by ritonavir and nelfinavir (protease inhibitors) and grapefruit juice. Their levels are reduced by rifampicin, some medicines used for treatment of epilepsy and steroids. It is not recommended along with rifampicin and some tranquillisers.

Zidovudine is recommended in almost all combinations of medicines recommended for treatment of HIV infection. This is because its benefits have been observed for a long time and it can enter the brain more effectively than other medicines. HIV not only affects the blood but can also enter the brain. Thus, if a medicine does not enter the brain, it cannot control the infection effectively.

It is important to remember that the above description of medicines is merely a guideline. There are several options for a combination of more than one medicine currently recommended for treatment of HIV infection. Their use is based on the initial findings of several studies. The understanding of the effect of these medicines and the most effective combination is changing rapidly. It is therefore desirable that the treatment is taken only from a doctor who is trained in the management of HIV/AIDS and has had experience of treating a large number of such cases.

How is the benefit of the treatment assessed?

Blood tests are normally recommended for assessing the benefit of treatment. In case the benefits are not as expected and the treatment regimen is proposed to be changed, a second test to estimate the number of HIV in the blood is recommended before changing the treatment.

If the treatment regime is to be changed, it is desirable that a complete new regimen is started. In case this is not possible, then at least two new medicines need to be added. It is not desirable to either change or add a single medicine to a treatment regimen that does not give the desired results.

In case the options for a new regimen are limited due to non-availability of medicines or side-effects or the need to take other medicines, it is desirable to continue the previous regime that has given partial results. If there is difficulty in tolerating one medicine, it may either be replaced with any other medicine or its dose be changed to a level that can be well tolerated.

What is the role of other systems of medicine management of HIV infection?

In India, majority of the people with HIV infection cannot afford or have access to the allopathic medicines recommended for treatment of HIV infection. A large number of people therefore seek treatment from practitioners of Indian systems of medicine or traditional healers. There have been several reports of successful treatment of HIV infection by a few practitioners of the Indian systems of medicine such as Ayurveda and Siddha.

Although most of these claims have not yet been proven, the Government of India has been supporting studies to test some of these medicines. There have been some initial success with some Ayurvedic and Siddha medicines (for example Immu-21) but further research is needed for definite indication on their effectiveness.

It is important that people with HIV infection do not seek treatment from unverified sources or traditional practitioners who promise them a definite cure. If specific treatment from Indian systems of medicine is preferred, it should be taken from a major government hospital where they are being studied scientifically. Also, seeking treatment from a major hospital will help detect opportunistic infections at the earliest and start appropriate treatment.

The key to effective treatment for HIV infection is early detection and intervention. This is because early treatment helps strengthen the immune

Box 8. Correct technique for using condoms

- Tear the tip of the condom packet making sure that you do not touch the condom with any sharp instruments or nails.
- Gradually slip the condom out of the packet by gently pressing the base of the packet.
- Hold the tip of the condom and place it on the tip of the erect penis. Unroll the condom. Holding the tip prevents air from being trapped inside the tip. It also allows some space for collecting the ejaculation fluid at the end of the sexual act.
- Withdraw from the sexual partner immediately after the ejaculation by holding the condom firmly to the base of the penis.

- Withdraw the penis from the condom making sure that the ejaculated fluid does not spill out.
- Wrap the condom in a piece of paper and discard it later in a dustbin.

Points to remember:
- Check the expiry date before buying condoms. Do not use the condoms after the expiry date is over.
- Store condoms in a cool and dry place where there is no exposure to direct sunlight. Do not store condoms in purse, back pockets of the pants, wallets or glove compartment of the vehicles.
- Do not use condoms if the packet is damaged.
- Use a new condom for every sexual act, irrespective of the type of sex.
- Wear the condom as soon as erection occurs and before any skin-to-skin contact takes place between the genital organs.
- In case there is a need for lubrication, use water- based lubricants only such as glycerine or lubricating jellies. Oil-based lubricants such as petroleum jelly, lotion, oils, etc., can make the condom weak.

system, reduces stress and allows lifestyle changes such as eating a well-balanced nutritious diet.

Complimentary systems such as Ayurveda, Homoeopathy, Unani, Nature Cure and Yoga can help reduce stress and maintain health. Several medicines recommended in these systems are believed to strengthen the immune system. Thus, even if the HIV infection cannot be cured, it can be controlled by making the immune system stronger and preventing opportunistic infections.

Before treatment is started from a practitioner of Indian systems of medicine, it is desirable that objective information about the therapy is obtained.

In addition to talking to the medical practitioner promoting the treatment, it is important to talk to people who have been treated by the same practitioner in the past, especially a few months or years before. Information on the advantages, disadvantages, side-effects and associated risks should be collected from all the available sources.

Extracts of some herbs used in Ayurveda and Nature Cure that are known to strengthen the body's natural defence mechanism are available as capsules or tablets. These include among others, aloe vera, liquorice, ginseng, St. Johnswort, etc. While the effectiveness of these herbs on the HIV infection is not yet known, they can help improve general health.

Severe stress is common among people with HIV infection. They are often isolated from the family and community and are not given the necessary care. Regular exercises in consultation with the medical practitioner, yoga, meditation, etc. can reduce stress levels and improve the quality of life. The exercise routine needs to be started in consultation with a medical practitioner.

What are the dietary recommendations for HIV infection?

Diet plays an important role in maintaining normal health. It is especially important for people who have HIV infection as poor nutritional status increases the risk of opportunistic infections. A balanced diet of cereals, proteins and large portions of vegetables are recommended for people with HIV infection.

Cereals contain complex carbohydrates, B-complex vitamins, proteins and several minerals. Since they are the main source of energy, they should form the major portion of the entire diet. Protein requirement for people with HIV infection is suspected to be higher than those without the infection. Proteins from eggs and dairy products are of good quality. Fish and meat can also be good sources of proteins. Vegetarians need to eat larger portions of whole grains, nuts and legumes to meet the daily protein requirement. Since the body does not store proteins, it is important that adequate proteins are consumed everyday.

Dairy products such as milk, yogurt, paneer, cheese, etc., are rich in calcium. Regular intake of these foods helps maintain normal functions of the muscles, bones, nerves and the brain.

Vegetables and fruits are also an important part of the balanced diet. They provide vitamins and minerals necessary for healthy living. Coloured vegetables and fruits (such as carrots, papaya, green leafy vegetables, etc.) are preferable because they have important nutrients such as beta carotenes. They are also important *anti-oxidants*, which are essential for maintaining normal health. Anti-oxidants are chemicals or other agents that inhibit or retard oxidation of a substance to which they are added. Oxidation is the term used for any process that increases oxygen content of a substance.

HIV infection increases the risk of wasting of the muscles. As a result, the affected person becomes weak and sick. In order to avoid muscle wasting, people with HIV need to exercise regularly and eat small and frequent meals everyday. Three meals and two snacks are desirable at fixed times. These meals should be taken even if there is no hunger.

Fluids such as water, fruit juices and herbal teas should be consumed more by people with HIV infection. Coffee and tea can lead to dehydration and therefore their intake should be limited to a total of about four cups a day. Alcohol should be avoided as it adversely affects the liver, especially if taken along with medicines.

What is the risk of occupational exposure to HIV?

Doctors, nurses, paramedical workers and other staff who work in any health care setting are at the risk of being exposed to HIV infection. This may be through injury from contaminated needles or sharp instruments or through contact of the eye, nose, mouth or the skin with infected blood. The risk through contact with infected blood is greater when the health care worker has cuts or wounds in his/her skin.

Several studies have indicated that most exposures for health care workers do not result in HIV infection. The risk of infection varies with the type of exposure and three main factors:

a. The amount of infected blood involved in the exposure;
b. The amount of virus in the infected blood at the time of exposure; and
c. Whether any medicines for HIV infection are taken after the accidental exposure.

The risk of getting HIV infection after a pin-prick with an infected needle or superficial cuts with infected sharp instruments is reported to be about 0.3 per cent. The risk after exposure of the eyes, nose or mouth to infected blood is about 0.1 per cent. The risk after exposure of the skin to infected blood is estimated to be less than 0.1 per cent. This risk is present only if there are cuts or wounds on the skin. So far no case has been reported of HIV infection through intact skin.

Most injuries with needles can be prevented by practising standard precautions (such as not recapping needle by hand) and by disposing used needles in suitable containers. Protective wear such as gloves, eye and face protection and gowns can prevent accidental exposure to eyes, mouth and skin.

What is the treatment for occupational exposure to HIV?

The place where the skin has been pricked by an infected needle or cut by a sharp instrument should be washed thoroughly with soap and water. In case the body fluids have splashed on the face, nose, mouth or skin, the parts should be flushed with water. If the body fluids have come in contact with the eyes, the eyes need to be flushed with clean water or saline solution.

Medicines for HIV infection are recommended after accidental exposure to the virus if the risk of getting the infection is very high. Common medicines recommended for occupational exposure to

HIV include zidovudine, lamivudine and a protease inhibitor, preferably indinavir. Zidovudine is recommended for treatment of all types of exposures involving HIV infected blood and other body fluids and tissues. Lamivudine given in combination with zidovudine increases its effectiveness and is recommended for virus that are resistant to zidovudine. This combination is safe if used for a short time.

Indinavir is added to the above two medicines only if the risk of exposure is very high, such as exposure to large volume of blood with a large number of HIV virus.

In case treatment for occupational exposure is desirable, it should ideally be started within one to two hours of exposure. Treatment may be started after longer periods of about one to two weeks in case of very high-risk exposure. In such cases, even if HIV infection cannot be prevented, the treatment can reduce the severity of symptoms and delay the progression of the disease.

The normal duration of treatment after occupational exposure is not known. Most medical practitioners however recommend treatment for about four weeks.

Information on taking medicines for preventing HIV infection after occupational exposure during pregnancy is inadequate. However, some studies have indicated that zidovudine can be taken after the fourth month of pregnancy.

It is important to remember that understanding of medicines used to control HIV infection is rapidly changing. This is why medicines should be taken only after consulting a doctor who has been trained in the management of HIV infections and who has had experience of treating several patients with HIV infection.

Follow up after occupational exposure to HIV infection is very important. The blood should be tested for HIV antibodies soon after exposure and every six weeks until six months after exposure. This is to detect the antibodies at the earliest in case there is an infection. In case medicines are taken for preventing HIV infection after occupational exposure, blood tests are recommended before starting the treatment and two weeks after. This is to check for any adverse reactions of the medicines.

In case there are any flu-like symptoms within three to four months after occupational exposure to HIV, it is important to be examined by a doctor trained in the management of HIV infection. This is because these flu-like symptoms such as fever, rash, pain in the muscles, tiredness or swollen lymph glands may indicate either HIV infection, reaction to medicines or other infections. A trained doctor will be able to recommend appropriate measures to identify the symptoms if they are because of HIV infection.

It is desirable that people avoid donating blood for about six to twelve weeks after occupational exposure to HIV. They should also use condoms for every sexual act in order to prevent transmission of infection to the sexual partner.

How can HIV/AIDS be prevented?

HIV/AIDS can be prevented in four main ways:
1. Being in a mutually faithful sexual relationship. If this is not possible, then correct and consistent use of condoms for every sexual act, irrespective of the type of sex is essential.
2. Checking all the blood and blood products for HIV infection before transfusion.
3. Avoiding drug abuse, especially injectable drugs. Sterilised needles and syringes should always be used for injections, especially intravenous injections.

4. Reducing the risk of mother-to-child transmission by giving appropriate treatment to a pregnant women who has HIV infection.

What are the benefits of using condoms?

Condoms greatly reduce the risk of getting infections such as sexually transmitted diseases and HIV/AIDS. They also prevent pregnancy. More than seventy-four per cent HIV infections in India are due to heterosexual route. Up to thirty-six per cent people attending special clinics for sexually transmitted diseases have been reported to have HIV infection. Thus, correct use of condoms for every sexual act is important for preventing sexually transmitted diseases including HIV infection. Many people use condoms only with non-regular sexual partners or when they are not sure of the 'health' and 'hygiene' of the partner.

This type of inconsistent use can increase the risk of getting infections. Anyone who has multi-partner sexual behaviour needs to use condoms for all sexual acts, including with the married partner.

Box 8 describes the steps in correct technique for using condoms. There are several myths related to the use of condoms. The facts related to these myths are described in Box 9.

Box 9. Common myths related to condom use

Myth: *Condoms are not effective.*

Fact: This is not true. Several studies have persuasively indicated that failure of prevention of pregnancy with condoms is often because of inconsistent and incorrect use of condoms. This is also true for sexually transmitted diseases including HIV/AIDS.

Myth: *Condoms often break during sexual act.*

Fact: This is not true. All latex condoms manufactured in India are tested for defects before they are packed. During the manufacturing process, several strict quality methods are adopted. Condoms normally break only if they have not been used correctly or have been damaged because of improper storage.

Myth: *Condoms do not protect against HIV because the virus can pass through the condoms.*

Fact: This is not true. Several studies have indicated that condoms act as a highly effective barrier against sperms and disease causing germs including HIV.

Myth: *Condoms reduce sexual pleasure.*

Fact: This is not necessarily true. There may be a difference in the sensation in the initial stages of using condoms but most people adapt to them very soon. Also, newer condoms such as ribbed condoms, dotted condoms, etc., are reported, to enhance pleasure for some people.

Myth: *Knowledge about using condoms promotes sexual activity among the young.*

Fact: This is not necessarily true. Several studies worldwide including in India have indicated that providing information on condoms does not influence sexual activity among young. Some studies have indicated that this knowledge helps young people to abstain from early sexual activities.

What are the different types of condoms?

There are several types of latex condoms available in India. All these condoms are lubricated in order to facilitate sexual activity. Condoms are available in a wide range of colours and flavours. Some condoms have ribbed or dotted surface that are reported to increase sexual pleasure. All the condoms manufactured by major condom manufacturers in India meet with international standards of condom quality.

A female condom prepared from polyurethane has recently become available in the United States of America. It is a vaginal pouch that acts as a mechanical barrier to viruses. More studies are needed to determine if the female condoms are effective in preventing transmission of HIV infection. Female condoms are not easily available in India and if available, are very expensive.

Recently, polyurethane condoms have also been manufactured in some countries. Studies are underway to determine if these condoms are as effective as latex condoms in preventing pregnancy and sexually transmitted diseases. Polyurethane condoms can be made thinner than latex condoms and may also be used with oil-based lubricants.

How can diseases be prevented in people with HIV infection?

Opportunistic Infections:
Since HIV infection increases the risk of several opportunistic infections, it is important to take special precautions to prevent them. Detailed below are the preventive measures for common opportunistic infections.

- **Sexually transmitted diseases:** Regular use of condoms for all sexual activities can prevent sexually transmitted diseases. It can also prevent infection with HIV virus. Condoms also prevent transmission of HIV infection to the sexual partner.

- **Injection drug use:** In India, about nine per cent people with HIV infection are reported to have acquired it through injection drug abuse. The risk is higher in states such as Manipur where the number of people using injection drugs is higher. Injection drug abuse also increases the risk of getting other infections such as hepatitis B and C infections. This is why people who abuse injectable drugs need to be counseled to stop using the drugs. Box 10 lists the precautions that are recommended for people who continue to inject drugs.
- **Infections:** People who work in health centres and hospitals or those who live in crowded places are at the higher risk of getting infections, especially major infections such as tuberculosis. It is advisable that as far as possible, people

Box 10. Recommendations for people who continue to abuse injectable drugs

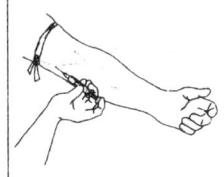

Efforts should be made to stop people from using injectable drugs. If these do not succeed, the following measures are recommended to prevent HIV infection.

- Do not share syringes, needles, water or equipment used to prepare drugs.
- Do not reuse needles that have been used by anyone for injecting drugs.
- In case injection equipment needs to be shared, it is important to first clean it with bleach and water.
- Use only sterile needles and syringes collected from a reliable source such as a pharmacy or a non-government organisation that implements needle and syringes exchange programmes.
- Use boiled water to prepare drugs. If it is not possible, use only fresh tap water.
- Use new cotton and disinfected container to prepare drugs.
- Clean the injection site with a new cotton swab dipped in alcohol.
- Dispose the syringes after one use in a safe manner or give them to agencies that are involved in needle and syringe exchange programmes.

with HIV infection should not work in places where they have higher risk of coming in close contact with tuberculosis patients.

Adults who take care of children are at greater risk of getting infections such as giardiasis, cytomegalovirus infection, etc. This risk is higher among people who work in paediatric wards of hospitals or child care centres. These infections can prevented by adopting good hygienic practices. It is desirable that hands are washed thoroughly clean after washing babies who have passed urine or stools.

People who work with farm animals such as cows, buffaloes, etc. are at higher risk of getting infections such as cryptosporidiosis and toxoplasmosis, especially if the animal has diarrhoea. Good hygiene such as hand washing after every contact with the animals can greatly reduce this risk. People with HIV infection should also avoid contact with their pet animals when they have diarrhoea in order to prevent opportunistic infections. They should also avoid getting new pets that are less than six months old or those that have not been examined by a doctor for any illness, especially diarrhoea.

- **Food and water-borne diseases:** Raw or undercooked food increases the risk of getting diarrhoea and other infectious diseases. This is why it is advisable that people with HIV infection avoid raw or under-cooked eggs, poultry and seafood. They should also avoid unpasteurised milk or dairy products. Uncooked foods should not be allowed to come in contact with cooked foods in order to avoid cross contamination of foods. Hands and all the utensils, cutting boards and knives used for cutting vegetables or preparing foods should be washed well after contact with uncooked foods. Cold or frozen foods should be consumed only after they have been heated till they are steaming.

Drinking water from sources whose safety cannot be guaranteed must be avoided. Most tap water in India from municipal sources is safe unless there is risk of contamination with sewage in the distribution channels. Water collected from a water purifier that uses "reverse osmosis" method is safe. Some of the disease-causing germs are very small and are therefore not removed by all filters. Information on the types of germs that the filter can remove can be obtained from the literature given with the filter or the manufacturers. In case of any doubt, only boiled water should be consumed. Filters need to be cleaned by a person who does not have HIV infection in order to prevent contamination of the hands while cleaning them.

It is advisable that people with HIV infection avoid swimming in lakes, rivers, etc., where the water is likely to be contaminated with human or animal wastes. This is because if they swallow water while swimming, they can get diarrhoea and other infections.

Aerated drinks in restaurants, bars, theatres or other public places should be avoided unless they are in sealed containers. Fountain drinks should also be avoided. Ice should not be added to any soft drinks or drinking water as it may be prepared from contaminated water.

Tuberculosis:

Tuberculosis (TB) is a disease caused by a germ called Mycobacterium tuberculosis. It normally affects the lungs, but can also infect other parts of the body. Tuberculosis may be latent or active. "Latent" means that the bacteria are in the body but do not cause any symptoms. People with latent tuberculosis cannot spread the infection to others. Since HIV infection weakens the body's natural defence mechanism, the bacteria can begin to multiply and cause active tuberculosis. This means that there will be symptoms. A person with tuberculosis can infect other people only if the infection is present in the lungs. A person with HIV infection and tuberculosis is said to have AIDS.

As mentioned earlier, the risk of getting tuberculosis infection increases in people with HIV infection who are working in hospitals and clinics. This is because they are at higher risk of coming in contact with people with active tuberculosis. As far as possible, people with HIV infection should therefore avoid coming in close contact with any person with active tuberculosis. They can be in contact with a person who has been taking medicines for a few weeks to cure tuberculosis.

Some medical practitioners recommend that people who have voluntarily tested for HIV infection and are positive should also be tested for tuberculosis. This is done through a skin test called *tuberculin test*. In this test, a small amount of testing fluid (called tuberculin) is injected just under the skin on the arm. The results are read after two or three days. In case the test result is positive, it indicates latent tuberculosis. In such cases, additional tests such as x-ray of the chest and examination of the sputum are normally recommended to detect active tuberculosis, if any.

In case the skin test is negative for tuberculosis, it is recommended that the test be repeated at least once a year, especially if there is a greater risk of getting the infection.

Some medicines are often recommended for people with latent tuberculosis in order to prevent it from becoming active. One of the most commonly used medicine is isoniazid along with a vitamin called pyridoxine to prevent *peripheral neuropathy*, a disorder of the nervous system.

This treatment is normally recommended for about twelve months because the tuberculosis bacteria die very slowly. Isoniazid is not recommended during the first three months of pregnancy.

In case isoniazid is not effective in preventing tuberculosis or is contraindicated, other medicines such as rifampicin are recommend to prevent active tuberculosis.

The medicines recommended for treatment of tuberculosis are the same for people with or without HIV Infection. There are several medicines and the doctor is the best person to decide the combination of medicines that is most likely to be effective.

The symptoms normally disappear a few weeks after starting the treatment but since the bacteria takes a long time to die, the treatment is recommended at least for about six to nine months.

Irregular treatment prevents complete cure of tuberculosis. It can also lead to drug resistance. This means that the bacteria are not killed by the medicines being taken. People who have drug-resistant tuberculosis can transmit the resistant bacteria to others.

This means that the person who has contracted the infection will also not respond to the medicines. When several medicines fail to kill the bacteria, the tuberculosis is called "multidrug-resistant" tuberculosis. In India, the number of people with drug resistant and multi-drug-resistant tuberculosis is increasing rapidly.

Detailed information on the different medicines recommended for treatment of tuberculosis, their recommended doses, duration of treatment and common side-effects can be discussed with the doctor or attending physician.

Cryptosporidiosis:

Cryptosporidiosis is caused by a parasite called Cryptosporidium parvum. Many people with cryptosporidiosis may not have any symptoms. If they do, the symptoms include watery diarrhoea, stomach cramps, or a slight fever. These symptoms appear about two to ten days after the person is infected.

Cryptosporidiosis can be serious and long-lasting in people with AIDS as they have a weak immune system. If the CD4+ count is above two hundred, the illness may not last more than one to three weeks. However, the infection can still be present and the symptoms may reappear when the CD4+ count drops below two hundred.

Since cryptosporidiosis is normally spread by oral route, good personal and food hygiene can prevent it. Washing the hands often with soap and water is important to prevent the infection. Hands should always be washed before eating and preparing food. They should also be washed after (a) touching clothing, bedding, toilets, or bed pans soiled by someone who has diarrhoea, (b) gardening (c) touching pets or other animals and (d) touching anything that might have had contact with even the smallest amounts of human or animal stool, including dirt in your garden and other places.

Cytomegalovirus:
This virus is found in all parts of the world. It can cause retinitis in a person with HIV infection or AIDS. The symptoms include blurred vision and blindness, pain while swallowing, diarrhoea, and pain, weakness, and numbness in the legs.

Cytomegalovirus spreads from one person to another through saliva, semen, vaginal secretions, blood, urine, and breast milk. When a person touches these fluids with hands and then touches his/her nose or mouth, cytomegalovirus can occur. It can also be transmitted through sexual contact, breast-feeding, blood transfusions, and organ transplants.

Cytomegalovirus can be prevented by washing hands frequently and thoroughly and using condoms. Most blood banks test blood for cytomegalovirus. The test is sometimes recommended for people with HIV infection who need a blood transfusion.

In recent times, some doctors in India have been reporting several cases of cytomegalovirus, especially retinitis. This infection does not always cause symptoms, especially in people with normal immune system. Occasionally, it may cause fatigue, swollen glands, fever, and sore throat but since these symptoms can also occur due to other illnesses, it is difficult to detect cytomegalovirus.

Penumocystis Carinii:

In countries such as the US, this is the most common serious infection among persons with HIV. It can be fatal. It is caused by bacteria called Pneumocystis carinii. Most people infected with these bacteria do not get pneumonia if their immune systems are normal. Pneumocystis carinii can be cured with medicines.

Exposure to pneumocystis carinii is difficult to prevent and therefore medical treatment is recommended to prevent the infection. The best drug for preventing pneumocystis carinii is trimethoprim-sulfamethoxazole, a combination of two medicines. This medicine is recommended if the CD4 cell count falls below two hundred or if there are symptoms such as fever and fungal infection in the mouth (oral thrush).

Toxoplasmosis:
People with HIV infection usually have symptoms because of toxoplasmosis if their CD4 count is below hundred. This infection normally affects the central nervous system, including the brain. Many people infected with toxoplasmosis have no symptoms. However, people with HIV or

AIDS may have symptoms such as headache, confusion, and fever. Other symptoms include seizures, poor coordination, and nausea.

Toxoplasmosis can be spread in two ways: (a) by eating under-cooked meat; and (b) through contact with infected cat stool. It can be prevented by eating meat that is cooked till it is no longer pink in the centre. Red meat is safe if it has been frozen for at least twenty four hours. Chicken and eggs almost never contain toxoplasmosis. However, they should also be cooked until well done because of risk of other diseases.

Box 11 lists the medicines recommended for treatment and prevention of some common opportunistic infections along with their doses and duration of treatment. Preventing opportunistic infections and their early diagnosis and treatment can improve the quality of life of people with HIV infection.

Box 11. Medicines recommended for opportunistic

Opportunistic disease	Medicines
Candidiasis	Ketoconazole Fluconazole Itraconazole liquid
Cryptococcosis (Acute treatment)	Amphotericin B Flucytosine Fluconazole
Cryptococcosis (Consolidation treatment)	Amphotericin Fluconazole Itraconazole
Cryptococcosis (Secondary prevention)	Fluconazole Amphotericin
Cytomegalovirus infection (Prevention)	Ganciclovir Ganciclovir Foscarnet Cidofovir
Cytomegalovirus infection (Treatment)	Ganciclovir Foscarnet Cidofovir
Herpes simplex and zoster	Simplex Aciclovir Zoster Aciclovir Encephalitis Aciclovir

treatment and prevention of common infections

Dose	Duration of treatment
200mg once a day	14 days
50mg once a day	7 days
100mg twice a day	7 days
1mg/kg daily	14 days
100mg/kg/day orally	14 days
800mg orally for 2 days followed by 600 mg daily	
1mg/kg daily	8 weeks
400 mg/kg	8 weeks
400 mg/day (liquid)	8 weeks
200 mg once a day	Long term
50 mg twice a week	Long term
1g 3 times a day orally	Long term
5mg/kg once a day	Long term
90 mg/kg once a day	Long term
5 mg/kg/14 days	Long term
5mg/kg 3 times a day	14 days
90mg/kg once a day	14 days
5mg/kg once a week	14 days
200 mg 5 times a day	5 days
800 mg 5 times a day	7 days
10mg/kg IV 3 times a day	10 days

Opportunistic disease	Medicines
Kaposisarcoma	Bleomycin 15 units and cincristine
Mycobacterium tuberculosis (Prevention)	Isoniazid
Mycobacterium tuberculosis (Treatment)	Rifampicin Isoniazid Pyrazinamide
Pneumocystis carinii pneumonia (Prevention)	Trimethoprim-sulfame-thoxazole Dapsone Dapsone with Pyrimethamine
Pneumocystis carinii pneumonia (Treatment)	Trimethoprim-sulfame-thoxazole Clindamycin and Primaquine
Toxoplasmosis (Treatment)	Sulfadiazine plus Pyrimethamine and Calcium Folinate Clindamycin plus Pyrimethamine and Calcium Folinate
Toxoplasmosis (Secondary prevention)	Sulfadiazine plus Pyrimethamine and Calcium Folinate Clindamycin plus Pyrimethamine and Calcium Folinate

Dose	Duration of treatment
2mg every three weeks	1 cycle
300mg daily	1 year
600mg once a day	6 months
300mg once a day	6 months
2g once a day	2 months
960mg once a day	Long term
100mg a day	Long term
100mg a day	
25 mg three times a week	Long term
90mg/kg/day	21 days
600mg four times a day	21 days
15 mg once a day	
2g three times a day	6 weeks
200mg in divided doses	
Followed by 50mg a day	
15mg a day	
600mg four times a day	6 weeks
200mg in divided doses	
Followed by 50 mg a day	
15mg a day	
1g three times a day	Long term
25mg once a day	
15mg once a day	
450mg three times a day	Long term
25mg once a day	
15mg once a day	

How can mother-to-child transmission of HIV infection be prevented?

Mother-to-child transmission is the most common source of HIV infection among children below fifteen years of age. About one million children are estimated to be living with HIV infection all over the world. Majority of these children are from the developing countries, especially Africa. Since HIV/AIDS is spreading rapidly in India, the number of pregnant women with HIV infection is also increasing. As a result, the number of children who get HIV infection through their mothers is also increasing.

Until recently, two main strategies were adopted to prevent mother-to-child-transmission of HIV infection. These included (a) to protect women in the childbearing age from becoming infected and (b) to promote family planning services in order to prevent unwanted births. Although these two strategies continue to remain the most important strategies for preventing mother-to-child transmission, a third option is being explored for reducing this mode of transmission. This is to give medicines that slow down the multiplication of HIV to pregnant women and sometimes to the infant too. In developed countries, breast-feeding is normally not recommended for babies born to mothers with HIV infection. However, the risk of ill health and death for a baby in countries such as India due to poor nutrition and diseases such as diarrhoea is much greater than the risk of getting HIV infection through breast-feeding. This is why all women in India, irrespective of whether they have HIV infection or not, are advised to breast-feed their babies.

One study in Thailand has indicated that taking a short-term treatment of zidovudine greatly reduces the risk of mother-to-child transmission. The risk is reduced to below ten per cent if breast-feeding is strictly avoided. However, in countries such as India where breast-feeding is important for prevention of infections such as diarrhoea for the infants, breast-feeding is recommended for all women, even if they have HIV infection. Some studies are underway to test whether a group of medicines are more effective than zidovudine. Initial reports of a study using zidovudine and lamivudine have shown promising results. More studies are underway to determine alternative medicines or groups of medicine that may further reduce the risk of mother-to-child transmission.

Some factors may increase the risk of mother-to-child-transmission of HIV Infection. The risk of transmission is estimated to be two times higher in a mother who has been recently infected with HIV as compared with a woman who has had earlier infection. This may be because of higher number of HIV in the blood after a recent infection. Vitamin A deficiency is also associated with increased risk of mother-to-child transmission. It is also suspected that fissures in the nipples of the mothers and oral thrush or wounds in the mouth of the babies increase the risk of mother-to-child transmission. This is because they allow the virus to enter the blood more easily.

Box 12 lists the risk factors associated with mother-to-child transmission.

Box 12. Factors that increase the risk of mother-to-child transmission of HIV infection

Strong evidence
Factors related to the mother
- Higher number of virus in the blood
- Type of virus
- Advanced stage of HIV infection
- Immune deficiency
- HIV infection acquired during pregnancy or breast-feeding period

Limited Evidence
- Vitamin A deficiency
- Anaemia
- Sexually transmitted disease
- Chorioamnionitis (Inflammation of the membranes covering the unborn child because of germs in the fluid surrounding the baby)
- Frequent unprotected sex*
- Multiple sex partners*
- Smoking
- Injecting drug use

*These increase the risk of the mother getting HIV infection

Factors related to type of delivery
- Vaginal delivery as compared with delivery through casesarean section)
- Prolonged rupture of membranes

- Invasive procedures such as forceps
- Episiotomy (Cut made in the perineum during delivery to enlarge the vaginal opening)

Factors related to the infant
- Premature birth
- Breast-feeding

- lesions of skin and/or mucous membranes (oral thrush)

How is HIV infection in children diagnosed?

HIV infection is difficult to diagnose in children. This is mainly because of two reasons. One, infected babies do not have any symptoms in the first few months and two, they have antibodies to HIV acquired from the mothers for up to eighteen months after birth. The tests to detect HIV antibodies cannot differentiate between antibodies passed on by the mother to the baby and those due to infection in the babies. Newer tests such as polymerase chain reaction (PCR) can detect small quantities of HIV virus in the infant's blood. Blood culture from a sample of the infant's blood can also be used to detect the presence of HIV. These two tests can detect about ninety per cent of infections in infants by two months of age and up to ninety-five per cent infection by three months of age.

What are the symptoms of children with HIV infection?

Many children with HIV infection do not gain the desired weight. They also tend to reach their milestones at a later stage as compared to uninfected children. As the disease progresses, the infected children can develop neurological problems such as difficulty in walking, confusion, lack of concentration, etc.

Just like adults, children infected with HIV are also at higher risk of getting opportunistic infections. Chronic diarrhoea and serious bacterial infections are more common among children with HIV infection than infected adults. These bacterial infections can cause fever, seizures, pneumonia, diarrhoea, dehydration and recurrent cold and cough. Most of these infections are serious enough to require hospital admission. Children with HIV infection also have severe candidiasis, a yeast infection. This infection can affect the mouth and throat and result in difficulty in swallowing. Toxoplasmosis is less common in children with HIV as compared to adults with the infection.

Pneumocystis carinii is one of the common causes of death in children with HIV infection. Cytomegalovirus infection is also more severe in children infected with HIV.

What is the progress of HIV infection in children?

About twenty per cent children with HIV infection develop serious disease in the first year of life. Majority of these children die by the age of four years. The remaining eighty per cent children have slower progress of HIV infection. These children may not develop serious symptoms until the age of six to seven years.

Factors that influence progress of HIV infection in children include levels of Vitamin A in the mothers during pregnancy, number of CD4 cells in the mothers during pregnancy and the number of HIV and CD4 cells in the baby during the first six months of life. It is believed that early treatment of babies with HIV infection can decrease the progression of the infection.

A large number of the medicines used to control HIV infection in adults are also recommended for infected children but in lesser doses. Several studies are underway to determine the most effective regimen to treat HIV infections in children with minimum side-effects.

Is there a vaccine to prevent HIV infection?

No, there is no vaccine currently available that can prevent HIV infection. Although several types of vaccines are in various stages of trial in developed countries, their effectiveness for prevention of HIV infection or to stop progression of the disease have not been conclusively proven. One of the main problems associated with development of vaccines against HIV is that the genetic composition of HIV is different in various parts of the world. Thus, a vaccine developed for a particular type of genetic composition will not be effective for other HIV viruses.

What are the ethical issues related to HIV infection?

HIV/AIDS is associated with severe social stigma and many people are forced to separate from their communities even after doing the first screening test for HIV. One positive result in a screening test in non-confirmation of HIV infection. Ethical issues related to HIV infection are mainly for ensuring that a person with HIV infection leads a life of dignity.

HIV testing should not be done without informed consent of the person to be tested. This means that the person to be tested should have understood what test results would mean and its likely impact on his/her life. Routine screening for HIV infection of all pregnant women and people needing surgery should not be done. The only exceptions to testing without taking informed consent are before donating blood or blood products and during routine surveillance. In both these situations the persons who test positive are not notified.

People with HIV infection have as much right to get medical treatment from any source as everyone else. It is unethical to deny medical treatment to a person with HIV or AIDS. Similarly, it is also unethical to deny employment to a person with HIV infection.

HEALTH UPDATE

YOUR PERSONAL MEDICAL ADVISOR

SOLUTIONS FOR ANY MEDICAL PROBLEM, AT YOUR FINGERTIPS

HEALTH UPDATE gives you detailed information on common diseases and ailments from five different perspectives- **Allopathy, Ayurveda, Nature Cure, Homoeopathy** and **Unani** in a concise and easy to understand format, complete with graphic descriptions, general information, health tips and much more.

SUBSCRIPTION

India ☐ 1 year-Rs. 300/- ☐ 2 years-Rs. 500/- ☐ 3 years-Rs. 750/-

International ☐ 1 year-$25 ☐ 2 years-$45 ☐ 3 years-$60

☐ Yes, I would like to subscribe to **Health Update**, the monthly health bulletin

Name: Mr./Ms..
Address (mention nearest landmark)..................................
....
City:................... State:.................... Country:....................
Pin:.................Tel:..................Fax:..............email:...............
Age/Profession..

☐ I am sending by Cheque/DD No..........................drawn on (specify bank)..................................... for Rs..................
dated......................... favouring **HEALTH UPDATE**.

☐ Please charge my American Express Credit Card

Credit Card No. ☐☐☐☐☐☐☐☐☐☐☐☐☐☐☐☐☐☐☐☐

Card Expiry Date.................Card Holder's Signature...........................

Date of Birth........................... Tel. (O) .... (R)..................

Direct this subscription form to:
HEALTH UPDATE, D-31, Defence Colony, New Delhi-110024, India.
Tel.: 4622863. Fax: 91-011-4698150. email: savitri_ramaiah@vsnl.com